Alkaline Juicing

The Easiest Way to Get Healthy and Feel Energized (Even If on a Busy Schedule)

The Alkaline Diet Lifestyle Series

By Marta Tuchowska

Copyright ©Marta Tuchowska 2018

www.HolisticWellnessProject.com

All rights reserved. No part of this publication may be reproduced, stored in a retrieval system, or transmitted, in any form or by any means, electronic, mechanical, photocopying, recording, or otherwise, without the prior written permission of the author and the publishers.

The scanning, uploading, and distribution of this book via the Internet, or via any other means, without the permission of the author is illegal and punishable by law. Please purchase only authorized electronic editions, and do not participate in or encourage electronic piracy of copyrighted materials.

All information in this book has been carefully researched and checked for factual accuracy. However, the author and publishers make no warranty, expressed or implied, that the information contained herein is appropriate for every individual, situation or purpose, and assume no responsibility for errors or omission. The reader assumes the risk and full responsibility for all actions, and the author will not be held liable for any loss or damage, whether consequential, incidental, and special or otherwise, that may result from the information presented in this publication.

The book is not intended to provide medical advice or to take the place of medical advice and treatment from your personal physician. Readers are advised to consult their own doctors or other qualified health professionals regarding the treatment of medical conditions. The author shall not be held liable or responsible for any misunderstanding or misuse of the information contained in this book. The information is not intended to diagnose, treat or cure any disease.

Contents

Introduction: Restoring Your Energy Levels with Plant-Based Foods and Alkaline Diet 9

Welcome to the World of Beautiful and Creative Alkaline Salads! 10

The Alkaline Diet - The Common Sense Approach .. 15

Alkaline Diet Crash Course - Understand the Basics (With No Pseudo-Science) 21

Your Free Gifts + Free Alkaline Newsletter 25

The Total Wellness Cleanse - Extra Recommendation by Marta 26

Alkaline Salad Recipes- Recommended Shopping List 28

Amazing Alkaline Salad Recipes 33

    Recipe Measurements 33

    Recipe #1 Tasty Thai Kale Salad 35

    Recipe #2 Stir-Fried Alkaline Vegetables 37

    Recipe #3 Miss Fresh Salad 39

    Recipe #4 Creamy Tasty Spicy Broccoli Salad 41

    Recipe #5 Healing Tomato Salad 43

    Recipe #6 Simple Celery Salad 45

    Recipe #7 Cherrying Apple and Celery Root Salad 47

    Recipe #8 Kale Mixed Up Salad 49

    Recipe #9 Greek-Style Bell Pepper Salad 51

Recipe #10 Gingered Pea Salad 53

Recipe #11 Radish Wakame Salad 55

Recipe #12 Super-Quick Parsley Salad 57

Recipe #13 Apple Pecan Tofu Salad 58

Recipe #14 Quick Quinoa Salad 60

Recipe #15 Arugula Lentil Salad with Lemon Parsley Dressing 62

Recipe #16 Olive Creation Salad 64

Recipe #17 Coconut Chickpeas with Roasted Broccoli Salad 66

Recipe #18 Smoked Tofu and Sweet Potato Green Salad 68

Recipe #19 Artichoke Dream 70

Recipe #20 Avocado Dream Salad 72

Recipe #21 Curry Love Quinoa Salad 73

Recipe #22 Tofu Salad with Mango and Avocado . 75

Recipe #23 Holiday Cranberry Buckwheat Salad .. 77

Recipe #24 Mediterranean Cilantro Chickpea Salad 79

Recipe #25 Coconut Quinoa Salad 81

Recipe #26 Hazelnut Banana Salad 83

Recipe #27 Roasted Asparagus Salad 84

Recipe #28 Kiwi Spinach Lentil Energizer 86

Recipe #29 Green Spicy Salad 88

Recipe #30 Buckwheat Salad with Spinach........... 90

Recipe #31 Watermelon Salad with Pecans and Cherries 92

Recipe #32 Plant-Based Greek Salad 93

Recipe #33 Summer Veggie Color Salad................. 95

Recipe #34 Green Papaya Dream Salad................. 97

Recipe #35 Green Orange Salad 99

Recipe #36 Yummy Grilled Zucchini Salad......... 101

Recipe #37 Happy Mizeria Salad......................... 103

Recipe #38 Fennel Salad with Tahini Coconut Dressing... 105

Bonus: Healthy Alkaline Salad Sauces and Condiments 107

Simple Alkaline Tahini Salad Dressing 107

Almost Alkaline Orange Dressing........................ 108

Chive Salad Dressing... 109

Alkaline Carrot Ginger Salad Dressing................. 110

Creamy Citrus Dressing 111

Italian-Style Tomato Cilantro Dressing 112

Catalina Almost-Alkaline Dressing...................... 113

Creating Your Alkaline Lifestyle for Energy You Deserve 114

Marta's Holistic Wellness Books............................ 116

Introduction: Restoring Your Energy Levels with Plant-Based Foods and Alkaline Diet

Do you bounce out of bed in the morning, or do you press the snooze button for just a few more moments of sleep? Can you get through the day without feeling fatigued?

Do you suffer from any ailments? Lack of energy? Can't lose weight even though you count calories and follow the latest "dieting" fads, making your life torture? I have been there too, and it wasn't until I discovered one simple solution that I could use to transform all areas of my health while enjoying higher energy levels and getting visible results. That solution is simple: it's a mix of healthy plant-based nutrition, an alkaline diet lifestyle, and holistic living. After making the transition, I never looked back. I also made it my mission to inspire and educate others on their journeys. This book, my other books in the Alkaline Diet Lifestyle series, and my blog, Holistic Wellness Project, are the fruits of my passion for making you passionate about a healthy lifestyle while making it easy, doable, and fun. I want to help you realize what works best for you and your beautiful body.

Welcome to the World of Beautiful and Creative Alkaline Salads!

First of all, thank you so much for taking an interest in this book, Alkaline Salads. It means a lot to me, and I am very excited for you as well. I know that the collection of recipes I am about to share with you will help you revolutionize your health and life in an easy and doable way.

Here's what I love most about alkaline salads:

1.They are quick and easy to make. Yes, some salad recipes from this book might take a bit longer to prepare, and you might want to save them for weekends, days off, or family occasions. But in most cases, it's easy peasy alkaline lemon squeezy, and you will love the convenience.

2.Recipes can be used as healing snacks (wow, isn't that a fantastic word combination? A snack that is fun and also helps us with healing?), as a separate meal, or as a side dish. This book doesn't tell you to live on salads. It encourages and inspires you to add more salads to your diet, specifically alkaline diet-friendly salads.

3.You can always add more ingredients to your salads if you choose to do so. Follow your instincts while combining ingredients. Make smart choices guided by your alkaline diet education, which you are investing in right now, and I am very excited for you because of that. I'm here to support you on your health journey.

My editor, Claire, is a 41-year-old professional woman who suffered from obesity, migraines, digestive problems, rashes, low immunity, and inflammation for many years. As a result of her overly acidic body stemming from the poor food choices she made, she experienced tremendous pain from gastric reflux, so much so that her doctor wanted to operate on her.

But once she started following an alkaline diet, she stopped having gastric reflux pain and began losing weight without feeling deprived. She found more energy and gets more done each day. She's happy with her new balanced lifestyle and suddenly has more energy and time to spend with her children. She keeps experimenting with new alkaline recipes and wants her family to eat healthily, too. She feels more productive with her work and can provide better services for her clients. And the best part is that she finally stopped counting calories! She loves eating, and she eats five times a day.

People who have changed their diets to an alkaline diet experience enormous benefits, and there are plenty of real-life stories to back it up. I, myself, have witnessed tremendous changes in my health; the alkaline diet combined with homeopathy, other natural therapies, and lifestyle changes helped cure my eye of uveitis (inflammation of the uvea, very often caused by autoimmune disorders), which is a serious eye disease that can even result in blindness.

I have also experienced a myriad of other benefits. That is why I am writing this book. I want to show you the practical way to alkalize your body with alkaline salad recipes so that you can FEEL it yourself.

To be honest with you, unlike other diets I have tried, the alkaline diet completely met my demands. I felt better and better every day physically, mentally and emotionally. The Alkaline Diet is the best holistic beauty treatment you can get.

It helps you glow. If you happen to have any skin problems or wish to 'look healthier,' the alkaline approach is the way to go.

High energy levels? You bet! I am brimming with energy. If you do the alkaline diet, your energy levels have no choice but to go up. I am an active person, and I love getting more and more stuff done. The alkaline lifestyle was one of the best things I have done for myself, and I just can't recommend it enough. All I had to do was learn how to add more alkalizing foods into my diet and how to reduce acid-forming foods. I had to go through a process of creating and organizing a new way of life. That is how I managed to burn excess fat and achieve my ideal weight without feeling deprived (I am a foodie!). I also feel stronger and hardly ever get colds or the flu. Even if I do, it's so mild that I don't feel affected at all and it goes away quickly.

Alkaline foods are for you if:

•You've tried dieting to lose weight and failed.

•You'd like to feel healthy and free of disease.

•You'd like to feel young and energetic again.

•You'd like to improve your skin.

•You'd like to stop being moody and irritated so often.

•You'd like to get rid of headaches, aches and pains, sinus issues, and insomnia.

•You'd like to improve your concentration and digestion.

The book you are reading right now focuses on practical tips and salad recipes. It is mostly for those who are already seasoned or have read my other books from the Alkaline Diet Lifestyle Series. However, it also stands on its own. So, even if this is the first time you are hearing about the Alkaline Diet, diving into the recipes and reading my additional tips will give you the tools you need to start transforming your lifestyle today. No fluff, no theory, and no complicated pH discussions. Just effective solutions that work and are easy to apply, even for busy individuals.

Additionally, I have three bonus PDF e-books for you and an incredible free newsletter to help you keep on track. It will help you live and enjoy the alkaline diet. Even if you already follow an alkaline diet, it will give you ideas for recipes and lifestyle tips.

Just visit the link below and follow the steps outlined to claim your free gifts and join our free newsletter to further help you on your journey:

www.holisticwellnessproject.com/alkaline

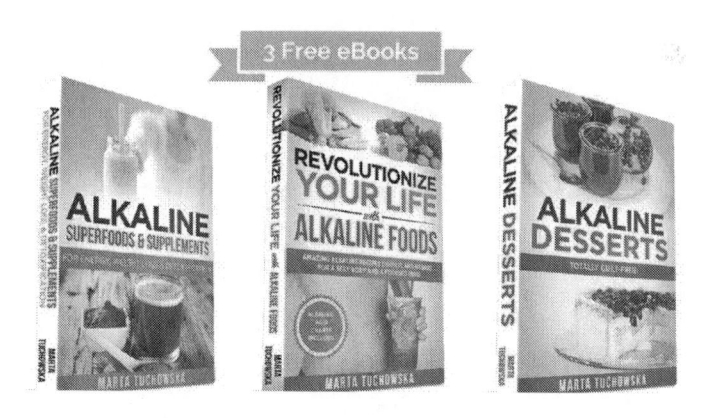

I recommend you grab them now before you forget. If you happen to have any questions about that process, simply email us at info@holisticwellnessproject.com.

Now, let's get into alkaline salads!

Here's our plan:

1.First, I will quickly explain the basic concepts of the alkaline diet and lifestyle with no pseudo-science or complicated jargon. That way, you will intuitively know where to shift your diet and lifestyle. (Part I)

2.Then, I will quickly guide you through some fundamental shopping lists to help you get organized faster. It is always my goal to create recipes that are easy to make and do not call for many fancy ingredients. However, I also like to use my recipes to educate my beloved readers, so if I call for any unusual ingredients, I will also try my best to explain what it is and what it does. I remember my frustration when I was transitioning into a healthy lifestyle and going through recipes that seemed like they were written in a new language. I know that can be frustrating, and I am doing my best to help you avoid frustration (hopefully). You can always reach out to me via my blog (HolisticWellnessProject.com) if you have any questions or doubts. (PART II)

3.Then, I will explain my best tricks to help you conjure up incredible alkaline salads and enjoy the process. That way, when you get into the recipes, not only will you feel more motivated and inspired, but you will also feel like it's very doable. (PART III) Then, in part IV, you will discover over 30 amazing salad recipes and a bonus section with healthy salad condiments. Easy peasy alkaline lemon squeezy!

Oh, that's the second time she's said "alkaline lemon," but aren't lemons acidic? It's time for some explanations. Thanks for your patience!

The Alkaline Diet - The Common Sense Approach

The alkaline diet is a lifestyle that encourages you to give your body the nourishment it needs so that it can work for you at its optimal levels without feeling too exhausted or acidic. Too much acidity in the body leads to depression, sickness, and obesity. It's very similar to the anti-inflammatory diet. In fact, the alkaline diet and anti-inflammatory diet are sisters.

What this means is that every disease, including excess weight, is caused by a body that is too acidic. Some things that can make your body too acidic are processed foods, sugar, gluten and yeast, meat and animal products, stress, alcohol, tobacco, drugs, caffeine, and pollution.

Luckily, the alkaline diet gives us natural tools to fix the problem. I am not talking about overpriced superfoods from overseas that are difficult to find and pronounce. The most straightforward methods are always the best, and you will be surprised by how healthy you feel by adding more everyday healing alkaline foods into your diet (even if you don't follow the alkaline diet strictly).

If you address the cause of the problem by implementing a lifestyle rich in alkaline-forming foods, it will naturally take care of what plagues you.

Here are a few guidelines that will help you transition towards a healthy alkaline lifestyle. These are compatible with different nutritional lifestyles (gluten-free, vegetarian, vegan), and it's entirely up to you what you choose to focus on:

1)Eliminate processed foods from your diet and say "no" to colas and sodas. There are copious additives and preservatives in these foods. They have been known to create hormone imbalances, make you tired, and add to acidity in your body. It's not natural for humans to consume those conveniently processed foods. The label may even say "low in calories" or "low in fat," but it will not help you in your long-term weight loss or health efforts. To start losing weight naturally, your body needs foods that are jam-packed with nutrients. Real, living foods. This, in turn, will help your body maintain its optimal blood pH (7.35) almost effortlessly.

2)Add more raw foods into your diet, especially vegetables, leafy greens, and fruits that are naturally low in sugar. Limes, lemons, grapefruits, avocados, tomatoes, and pomegranates are alkaline-forming fruits.

3)Reduce or eliminate animal products. These are extremely acid-forming. The good news is that there are many plant-based options out there and tons of ways to create delicious alkaline-friendly and plant-based meals that you will love! If I can do it, you can do it, too.

4)Drink plenty of clean, filtered water, preferably alkaline or fruit-infused water.

5)Add more vegetable juices into your diet. These are a great way to give your body more nutrients and alkalinity that will result in more energy, less inflammation, and if desired, natural weight loss. Vegetable juices are the best shots of health! I have also written a book called "Alkaline Juicing" if you want to give it a try and juice the right way.

6) Reduce or eliminate processed grains, "crappy carbs," and yeast. Again, these are very acid-forming. Personally, I recommend quinoa instead (naturally gluten-free), amaranth (super nutritious), brown rice, or soba noodles (made from buckwheat and naturally gluten-free). You can also use gluten-free wraps or make your own bread. Fruit is also an excellent natural source of carbohydrates and is great for energy. Plus, fruit always makes a great snack!

7) Reduce or eliminate caffeine. Trust me, it will only make you feel sick and tired in the long run and can even lead to adrenal exhaustion (not the best condition to end up in - I have been there). It may seem a bit drastic at first, and yes, I know what you're thinking, there are so many articles out there praising the benefits of caffeine and coffee. Yes, I am sure there are, and that's because many people build their business around coffee. That is why there must be something out there that promotes it. At the same time, I agree that everything is good for you in moderation.

As long as you have a healthy foundation, you can have coffee as a treat (I do drink coffee occasionally). There is no reason to be too strict on yourself, but don't rely on caffeine as your primary source of energy.

Green tea may be helpful as a transition, but green tea is not caffeine-free either, so don't overdo it. On the other side of the spectrum, green tea is rich in antioxidants and is an excellent part of a balanced diet, so you don't have to get paranoid about having caffeine. Moderation is the key.

Try to observe your body. I have noticed that quitting my coffee habits (I used to have 2-3 cups of coffee a day) and replacing coffee with natural herbal teas and infusions have made my energy levels skyrocket.

Now I sleep better, and I wake up feeling nice and refreshed. I don't need caffeine to keep me awake. I no longer suffer from tension headaches and feel calmer. Yes, I have a cup of coffee as a treat sometimes, usually when I meet with a friend, but I no longer depend on it. I choose it; it doesn't choose me. Think about this and how you can apply this simple tip to your life to achieve total wellbeing. Coffee and caffeine, in general, are extremely acid-forming.

I recently started using an Ayurvedic herb called ashwagandha. It is known as an adaptogenic herb, and it can help you restore your energy levels naturally. I highly recommend you give it a try!

8)Replace cow's milk with almond milk, coconut milk, or any other vegan-friendly milk, for example quinoa milk, chia seed milk, oat milk—whatever works well for you and your stomach. Cow's milk is exceptionally acid-forming, and personally, I don't think it makes sense for humans to drink milk that is naturally designed for fattening baby calves and not humans. Quitting dairy was one of the best things I have done for myself. I noticed that even just a little milk would cause digestive problems, and it was easy to fix—I quit drinking milk. I also learned about the cruelty in the dairy industry, which obviously contributed to my decision. The best thing about the alkaline plant-based diet is that you can still have ice cream and other treats, but you can make them without milk or animal products. It's so much healthier, tastier, and guilt-free. With this approach, there is no need to go hungry or deprived. You focus on the abundance of foods and meals that are both good for you and delicious, and that choice is also better for animals and the planet. That is what I call holistic motivation.

9)Don't fear good fats. Coconut oil, olive oil, avocado oil, etc. are good for you and should replace processed margarine and artery-clogging trans-fats. That is not to say that you can "drink" them freely. Balance is the key.

Use stevia instead of processed sugar (stevia is sweet but sugar-free) and Himalayan salt instead of regular salt. Himalayan salt contains calcium, iron, potassium, and magnesium, plus it also includes lower amounts of sodium than iodized salt.

Add more spices and herbs to your diet. Not only do they make your dishes taste incredible, but they also have anti-inflammatory properties and help you detoxify. Cilantro, turmeric, and cinnamon are miraculous.

As you can see, the alkaline diet is a pretty common-sense clean diet. Nothing is exaggerated. Nothing is too strict or faddish. Eat more living foods and avoid processed foods. Try to eat more plant-based foods. Don't reject it before you have tried it.

Add regular relaxation techniques to the alkaline diet including yoga, meditation, time spent in nature, adequate sleep, and physical activity (we need to sweat out those toxins), and you have a prescription for health. It's strange to me that there are so many people putting the alkaline diet down. However, the general guidelines I mentioned are common sense for a healthy lifestyle, and I am sure your doctor would agree with more natural foods, less processed crap, more relaxation, and less stress. This is the gist of the alkaline diet lifestyle.

This is what will make you feel healthy and rejuvenated and will help you achieve your ideal weight. The problem is that some people are not willing to take those small common sense steps and are looking for a "secret formula" or something that will magically help them with no effort at all. I am not judging—I have been guilty of it as well. We all have!

The truth is that whatever change you want to make in your life (this rule doesn't just apply to health) can be challenging because leaving one's comfort zone is difficult, but with time and practice, it becomes easy and automatic. Holistic success is about applying what we already know and using the information to better our lives. This is what I call "the secret formula." It's information in action.

I always say that I am very open-minded when it comes to different diets. I never claim that what I do is the only path to wellness and health. I prefer providing you with information and inspiration so that you can create your unique way and choose what works for you. Everyone is different.

You need to learn to listen to your body and be good to yourself.

Now, with that being said, try to adhere to the following recommendations - they will help you understand the alkaline diet without overwhelming you with complicated pH discussions.

You can easily get started today just by making some minor adjustments to your existing diet. Remember, take baby steps. I always try to make things simple and easy to apply. Once you apply it, you will feel the incredible benefits of alkalinity, and from there, you will want to carry on.

The alkaline diet is not a diet, but a lifestyle. It encourages you to add more alkalizing foods and drinks into your diet so that your body can heal itself naturally. How?

Alkaline Diet Crash Course - Understand the Basics (With No Pseudo-Science)

The pH of most of our fundamental cellular and other fluids like blood is designed to be at pH of 7.35, which is slightly alkaline.

The body has an intricate system in place to maintain that healthy, slightly alkaline pH level no matter what you eat. This is an argument that many alkaline diet skeptics use, and I get it. It's 100% true, and I say the same thing.

This is not the goal of the alkaline diet. We can't just make our blood's pH more alkaline or "higher." Our body tries to work hard for us to help maintain our ideal pH (7.35). We can't have a pH of 8 or 9. If we did, we would be dead.

The focus of the alkaline diet is to give your body the nourishment and healing tools that it needs to MAINTAIN that optimal 7.35 pH almost effortlessly.

If we fail to do so, we torture our body with incredible stress! Yes, when the body has to continually work overtime to detoxify all of the cells and maintain our pH, it finally succumbs to disease.

Let me name a few examples of what can happen if we continuously eat an acid-forming diet (also called SAD - Standard American Diet) that is not supporting our body at all. Our body ends up sick and tired of working overtime and may manifest one or more of the following conditions:

- Constant inflammation

- Immune and hormone imbalance

- Lack of energy and mental fog

- Yeast and candida overgrowth

- Digestive damage

- Weakened bones. Our body is forced to pull minerals like magnesium and calcium from our bones to maintain the alkaline balance it needs for its constant healing processes.

In summary, eating more alkaline foods helps support our body so that it can work for us at optimal levels while eating more acidic food doesn't help at all. The alkaline diet is not about magically raising our pH but helping our body rebalance itself by supporting its natural healing functions.

Why is it called an alkaline diet, then?

To be honest, I don't know. It could also be called the Eat More Veggies diet, or perhaps the Veggie Lover Diet, but then most people would never even look at it. I guess it was called the alkaline diet for a reason, probably to make it more mysterious and sexy so that there is this "hook" that makes people think, "Hmmm, what is it? That stuff must be hot!"

The alkaline diet is the sister of the clean food diet, anti-inflammatory diet, vegetarian diet, vegan diet, macrobiotic diet, and raw food diet. In fact, it offers an incredible blend, and best of all, all of those diets are in the plant-based diet category.

However, it's not just about what we eat. It's also about how we live and what we think. It's not just a diet; it's a lifestyle. If you want vibrant health and alkaline wellness, try to go outdoors more. Meditate, laugh, spend time with family and friends, do things you enjoy so that you can de-stress, and practice mindfulness. It's not just about nutrition; it's about your lifestyle.

Over the years, I have also learned that obsessing too much about food or health can be bad. You see, when you are too strict on yourself, this attitude saps your emotional wellness. Balance is the key. We don't want to be too rigid or obsessed, but we don't want to end up being too lenient, either. You need to be honest with yourself and ask yourself what you can do better. Reclaim responsibility for your health and wellness. It's always great to look for that next level. However, it's also good to cultivate the sense of gratitude and accomplishment for what we have already managed to change in our diets and lifestyles. Keep learning new recipes and gaining more information about alkaline, vegan, and plant-based lifestyles. Just keep moving forward, and you will get there. Trying is winning!

Often, it's not about eating less, but about eating right.

Your Free Gifts + Free Alkaline Newsletter

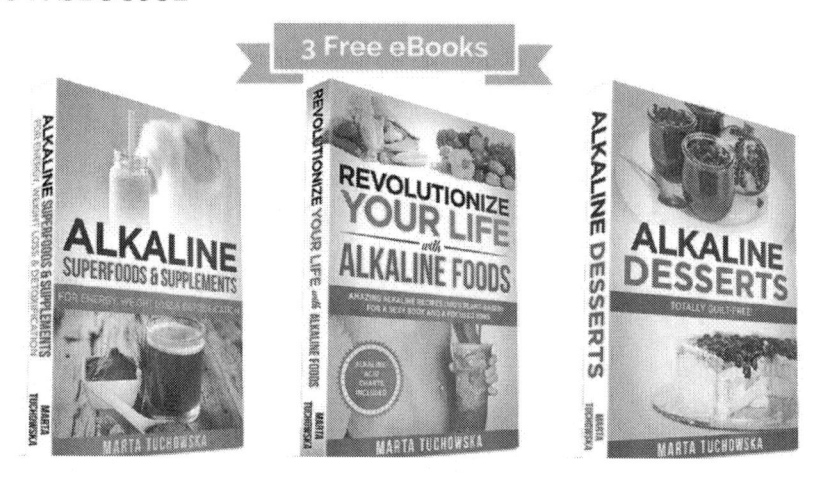

www.HolisticWellnessProject.com/alkaline

Never heard of the Alkaline Diet and don't know where to start?

I remember when I first learned about the alkaline diet. I was beyond confused and skeptical. I wanted to take action, but I didn't know how. I would spend endless hours online looking for alkaline-acid charts only to find that there was way too much contradictory information out there.

I don't want you to feel confused. I also appreciate the fact that you took an interest in my work. That is why I would love to offer you three free alkaline diet and lifestyle eBooks and easy alkaline-acid charts that are printable so that you can keep them on your fridge or in your wallet. They will provide a solid foundation to kick-start your alkaline diet success. You will get all the facts explained in plain English with practical alkaline tips and yummy vegan-friendly recipes full of taste, motivational advice, and printable charts for quick reference.

Visit:

www.holisticwellnessproject.com/alkaline

and follow the instructions to grab them now!

If you happen to have any problems, write us at:

info@holisticwellnessproject.com

The Total Wellness Cleanse - Extra Recommendation by Marta

Readers always ask me how I successfully transitioned to an alkaline-friendly clean food diet. It's very simple. Back in early 2013, I was a student of nutrition. However, the funny thing was that even though I was studying all those wonderful theories, I did not feel like I was eating healthy enough. Like most people out there, I had no idea what to eat. I mean, I was eating healthy compared to most of my friends, but I knew there was something better out there. I just had no clue how to put it all together in a simple, practical way that was easy to follow. I also felt tired, and because of that, it was hard for me to focus, think, concentrate, and transform my lifestyle. I was on the verge of giving up. Luckily, a friend of mine sent me a video by a gentleman named Yuri Elkaim. She recommended his program called the Total Wellness Cleanse. I was a bit skeptical at first. After all, there are so many online health scams going on, but I decided to give it a try. I absolutely loved it. It helped me properly transition to an alkaline diet because all I had to do was to follow his recommendations. Since I felt the results, I felt more motivated as well, and thanks to that program, I learned many interesting plant-based recipes.

Now, this is optional and beyond the scope of my book, but I want to quote it here as an additional recommendation to help you on your health and wellness journey if you choose to use it. On my blog, I wrote a very detailed article where I also shared my experiences and lessons learned with this program. I still use it a couple of times a year and recommend it as much as I can.

So, if you are looking for some extra resources, please don't hesitate to check out the article on my blog where you can learn more about it (feel free to post a comment below the blog post if you happen to have any questions about this program and the alkaline diet in general):

www.HolisticWellnessProject.com/alkaline-cleanse

Now, back to the salads! It's time to prepare for some massive wellness!

Alkaline Salad Recipes- Recommended Shopping List

Opt for fresh and organic fruits and vegetables. Order items online to save time or visit your local farmers' market. You can also order extra and split it with your neighbors and family to cut down costs. When it comes to fruits and vegetables, the fresher they are, the better. You can also start growing your own.

ALKALINE INGREDIENTS

These ingredients are super alkaline. I suggest you make them your priority.

Here's the list of HIGH alkaline foods.

Alkaline Veggies:

- Beetroot
- Capsicum or pepper
- Cabbage
- Celery
- Chives
- Collard and spring greens
- Endive
- Garlic
- Ginger

- Lettuce
- Mustard greens
- Onion
- Radish
- Red onion
- Rocket or arugula
- Wakame seaweed
- Spinach and kale
- Asparagus
- Carrot
- Courgetti or zucchini
- Leeks
- Pumpkin
- Squash
- Watercress
- Cucumber

These are NEUTRAL alkaline foods and can also be used in your salads:

- Cantaloupe
- Fresh dates
- Nectarine
- Plum

- Sweet cherry (Black Cherry)
- Watermelon
- Brazil nuts
- Pecans
- Hazelnuts
- Grapeseed Oil

Super Alkaline-Forming Fruits:

- Avocado
- Tomato
- Lemon
- Lime
- Grapefruit
- Fresh Coconut
- Pomegranate

Other Alkaline Salad Ingredients you might need:

- Herbs (basil, cinnamon, coriander, curry, rosemary, mint, thyme, etc.)
- Almond milk
- Coconut water
- Coconut milk

OILS:

Don't forget about oils- these are "good oils":

- Avocado oil
- Coconut oil
- Flax oil
- Udo's oil
- Olive oil

Alkaline nuts and seeds for more nutrients in your salads:

- Almonds
- Coconut
- Flax seeds
- Pumpkin seeds
- Sesame seeds
- Sunflower seeds

If you are pressed for time, resort to these to keep you energized:

- Himalayan salt (Contains magnesium, iron, and other vital minerals, and you can use it to give your smoothies and soups more flavor.)
- Cucumber
- Kale
- Kelp

- Spinach (baby or grown)
- Parsley
- Broccoli
- All kinds of sprouts (soy, alfalfa, etc.)
- Sea vegetables (kelp)

In case you forgot, you can get detailed and printable charts at: www.holisticwellnessproject.com/alkaline

Amazing Alkaline Salad Recipes

Recipe Measurements

Why is this European girl using American measurements?

It's simple. I am a big fan of making things easy. Life is already complicated enough. I love keeping ingredient measurements as simple as possible, and that is why I stick to tablespoons, teaspoons, and cups. You see, when it comes to making salads, you don't need to be that precise. What matters is your time and keeping it simple.

The cup measurement I use is the American cup measurement. I also use it for dry ingredients. If you are new to it, let me help you:

If you don't have American cup measures, just use a metric or imperial liquid measuring jug and fill it with your ingredient to the corresponding level. Here's how to do it:

1 American cup= 250ml= 8 fl. oz.

For example:

If a recipe calls for 1 cup of almonds, simply place your almonds into your measuring jug until it reaches the 250 ml or 8 oz. mark.

Easy, right?

I hope you found this helpful. I know that different countries use different measurements and I wanted to make things simple for you. I have also noticed that very often those who are used to American cup measurements complain about metric measurements and vice versa. However, if you apply what I have just explained, you will find it easy to use both.

Now, let's get into recipes. That's why we are here, right?

Recipe #1 Tasty Thai Kale Salad

Most people are not naturally attracted to kale. I wasn't until I found some delicious and exciting ways to adding kale into my salad, this recipe being one of them.

Kale is rich in vitamin K, vitamin C, vitamin A, manganese, and copper, as well as vitamin B6, fiber, calcium, potassium, and vitamin E (the list goes on and on), which makes it an extremely alkaline-forming ingredient.

And with this salad, it will be so easy to fall in love with kale. It's a raw, plant-based, nutrient-packed, beautiful salad that will help you energize your body and mind and feel amazing.

Nori gives salads an incredible twist and it also brings an incredible amount of nutrients to the table, for example vitamin C, potassium, vitamin a, and magnesium.

Serves: 1-2

Ingredients:

- 1 cup of kale leaves, stemmed
- ½ an onion (preferably red), thinly sliced
- Juice of 1 lime
- ½ cup organic coconut milk, thick (can be also coconut cream)
- 2 jalapeño peepers, diced
- Zest of 1 lime
- 2 orange or red bell peppers, diced

- 1 garlic clove, peeled, thinly sliced
- 1 avocado, peeled, pitted and sliced
- 1-2 nori sheets, soaked and chopped
- Himalayan salt to taste
- 2 tablespoons coconut oil
- Fresh coriander leaves to garnish

Instructions:

1. First, sauté the red onion slices in some coconut oil. Add the bell peppers, garlic, and jalapeño slices to the onions. Stir-fry until fragrant. Then set aside to allow to cool down.

2. In the meantime, chop the kale leaves. Place in a salad bowl and mix the lime zest and juice with the coconut milk. You can use your hands to make sure the kale leaves are thoroughly coated in the lime and coconut milk mix. Sprinkle over some Himalayan salt. Set aside.

3. Add the sautéed vegetables and avocado slices.

4. Add nori.

5. Toss well. Sprinkle over some coriander leaves, and if desired, serve with a slice of lime. Enjoy!

Serving suggestions: You can have this salad on its own, and it's perfect for a hot summer day. It also works as a standalone snack. It's rich in good fats from avocado and strangely enough will help you overcome unwanted sugar cravings.

I have also tried this salad alongside some curries, and it's a wonderful combination.

Recipe #2 Stir-Fried Alkaline Vegetables

There's nothing more delicious and nutritious than quinoa. Combine it with alkaline vegetables and you get an energy-filled lunch.

Serves: 1-2

Ingredients:

- 1-2 tablespoon coconut oil
- 1 big zucchini, chopped or spiralized
- 2 red bell peppers, chopped
- 1 small onion, roughly sliced
- 1 garlic clove
- 2 carrots (spiralized)
- 4 tablespoon cashew powder
- 1 cup (250g) cooked quinoa
- Himalayan salt to taste
- Juice of 1 lime
- Handful of cilantro
- Cumin powder (optional)

Instructions:

1. First, wash and spiralize the zucchini. Stir-fry in coconut oil (low heat), adding some Himalayan salt and a pinch of black pepper and cumin (optional, but I love it!) to taste. If you don't have a spiralizer, just finely chop the zucchini the way you want.

2. In the meantime, spiralize the carrots and chop the bell peppers, onions, and garlic. Keep an eye on the zucchini, you only want to stir-fry it until soft.

3. Set aside the zucchini and allow it to cool. In the meantime, in a salad bowl, mix all the ingredients (bell peppers, onion, garlic, quinoa, and carrots).

4. Mix in the zucchini, then sprinkle over some fresh lime juice, cilantro leaves, and Himalayan salt to taste. Finally, sprinkle over some fresh cashew powder. Enjoy!

Recipe #3 Miss Fresh Salad

This salad is perfect if you are looking for refreshment and revitalization. The recipe is very simple and effective, and is extremely alkaline-forming because of greens packed with vital nutrients that your body will be utterly grateful for.

Serves: 1-2

Ingredients:

- 4-5 iceberg or Romanian lettuce leaves
- 1 avocado, peeled, pitted and sliced
- 2 ripe tomatoes, finely sliced
- 1 garlic clove, peeled and finely chopped
- 1 cucumber
- 1 cup arugula leaves
- 1 orange, peeled and sliced
- 2 nori sheets, soaked
- Handful of parsley to garnish
- Some Himalayan salt to taste
- A pinch of black pepper
- Juice of 1 lime
- Handful of almonds
- 1 tablespoon olive oil

Instructions:

1.Mix all the ingredients in a salad bowl.

2.Add lime juice and toss well to make sure the lime juice is thoroughly spread.

3.Drizzle over some olive oil and add Himalayan salt and black pepper to taste.

4.Enjoy!

Recipe #4 Creamy Tasty Spicy Broccoli Salad

Why? What have I done to be punished with broccoli? My guess is that most people are not naturally attracted to broccoli. Well, this is where Marta Wellness comes in to help you spice it up and create an amazingly tasty and creamy salad that will make you forget the broccoli is even there.

Serves: 1-2

Ingredients:

- 1 cup of broccoli florets, chopped and slightly cooked
- ½ cup of green olives, sliced
- ¼ cup pistachios
- 2 mini cucumbers, peeled and diced
- Handful of raisins
- ½ an onion, sliced
- 4 tablespoons of vegan mayonnaise
- Juice of 1/2 a lemon
- 1 yellow bell pepper, finely chopped
- 1 orange bell pepper, finely chopped
- ¼ teaspoon Chili powder to taste
- Himalayan salt to taste
- ¼ teaspoon of black pepper
- 4 tablespoons thick coconut milk or coconut cream

- 2 slices of lemon or lime to garnish

Instructions:

1.In a salad bowl, place broccoli florets, green olives, pistachios, cucumbers, raisins, onions, and bell peppers. Drizzle over some lemon juice and Himalayan salt (one pinch) and toss well.

2.Now, mix the following ingredients in a small glass or bowl: vegan mayo, coconut milk or cream, black pepper, chili powder, and a pinch of Himalayan salt. Mix well.

3.Spread the mix onto your salad and garnish with 2 slices of lime or lemon (easy peasy alkaline lemon squeezy). Suggestion: Spread the salsa mix in the shape of a heart, because you deserve it! Mindful eating and self-love. Oh, and alkaline salads!

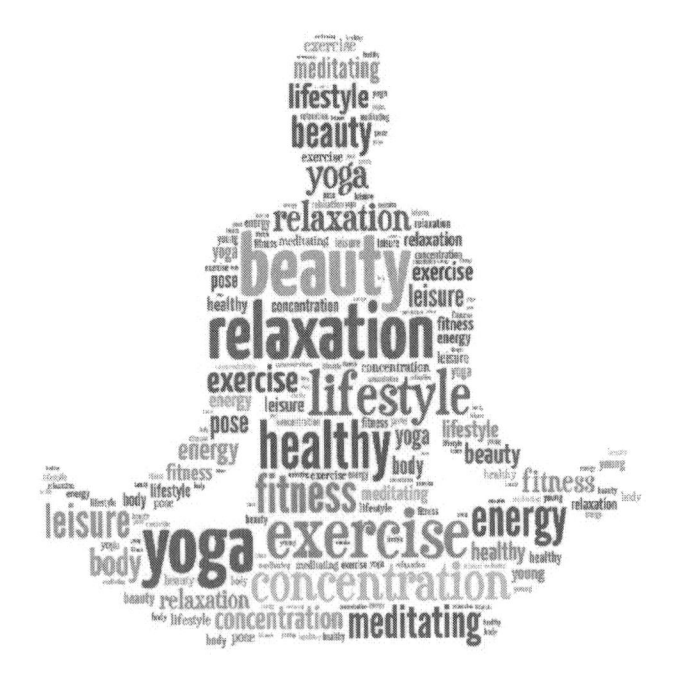

Recipe #5 Healing Tomato Salad

To get the most out of this recipe, I highly recommend you go for fresh organic tomatoes.

Did you know that the tomato is a fruit and not a veggie?

Many people do not give it enough credit. While looking for some expensive superfoods from overseas, we might forget about what's easily accessible and also very good for us. Tomatoes offer a variety of alkaline nutrients such as vitamin E, thiamin, niacin, vitamin B6, folate, magnesium, phosphorus and copper. They're also a source of dietary fiber, vitamin A, vitamin C, vitamin K, potassium, and manganese to help you alkalize your body, stay hydrated, and enjoy higher energy levels.

They can be added to your salads in a myriad of different ways while offering quick refreshment, energy boost, great taste, and alkaline-forming benefits (giving your body the vital nutrients it needs to pay you back with high energy levels).

Spinach and greens offer iron and chlorophyll while fresh orange juice adds to the vitamin C army. The original taste of this suburb healing salad will help your body function at its best!

Serves: 1-2

Ingredients:

- 2 large carrots, peeled and sliced (or spiralized)
- 4 large tomatoes, sliced
- Pinch of red chili

- 1 orange, juiced
- 1 medium garlic clove, chopped
- Pinch of black pepper
- Handful of fresh basil leaves
- Handful of fresh baby spinach leaves
- Handful of arugula leaves
- Handful of fresh parsley
- A few fresh mint leaves to garnish
- A few orange or mandarin slices to garnish
- 1 tablespoon of olive oil
- A pinch of Himalayan salt
- 1 teaspoon fresh oregano

Instructions:

1. In a salad bowl, place sliced tomatoes, garlic, and greens (spinach, arugula, parsley and basil).

2. Sprinkle over some fresh orange juice. Toss well.

3. Sprinkle on some Himalayan salt, red chili, and black pepper. Toss again. This process is to ensure that each leaf mixed into your salad has good flavor and there are no "bland surprises."

4. Now, place the spiralized carrots on top and sprinkle on some oregano. Garnish with fresh mint leaves and a few slices of orange or mandarin. Enjoy!

Recipe #6 Simple Celery Salad

Celery? In a salad? Is it a good idea? What will it taste like?

Have no fear. This salad offers a unique flavor, it's perfect for a quick aperitif, and it's great for people who don't like greens. Greens and the alkaline diet usually go together, or at least that is what you might remember from all the alkaline diet resources. And yes, there is definitely some connection, but the alkaline diet is not just about greens.

There are many other fantastic green foods that offer alkaline-forming benefits. Remember that simple rule? Whatever offers a myriad of nutrients, is low in sugar, and is a plant-based food (oh, and is gluten and yeast-free) is considered alkaline because it gives your body what it needs to reboot itself.

Again, it's a plain food, and it's easily accessible but often forgotten about by all the hot superfoods everyone talks about.

Serves: 1-2

Ingredients:

- 1½ cups of celery, spiralized (or sliced)
- 2 small carrots, spiralized (or sliced)
- Handful of fresh coriander
- 1 ½ tablespoons of vegan mayonnaise (can be replaced by coconut cream with some Himalayan salt)
- 1 tablespoon of chives (minced)
- ½ teaspoon of fresh organic lemon juice
- Sea salt to taste

- 3 tablespoons raw raisins
- A pinch of black pepper

Instructions:

1. In a salad bowl stir and mix the vegan mayonnaise with lemon juice, sea salt, and black pepper.

2. Add in the celery and carrots. Stir well.

3. Now sprinkle on some raisins, chives, and fresh coriander. Enjoy!

Recipe #7 Cherrying Apple and Celery Root Salad

Our recent salad hero, celery, is back again, this time accompanied by apples. An apple a day will keep the doctor away, as they say. While not considered strictly alkaline fruits, apples offer a myriad of nutrients such as vitamins A and C.

Also, they are fantastic for beginners and people who might still be having a hard time with veggies but have an easier time with fruits. All steps and habits on this journey are important, and I am always very happy to support you in all of your transformations. Let the old "one apple a day" shine in this salad (without outshining our buddy celery; he might get offended).

Serves: 1-2

Ingredients:

- 1 medium red apple (skin optional), diced
- 1 cup celery, peeled and sliced
- 4 tablespoons of chopped almonds
- Half cup cherries, pitted
- A few dates
- Juice of half a grapefruit
- Juice of half a lemon
- 2 tablespoons of coconut cream
- ¼ cup of minced fresh mint leaves

Instructions:

1. In a salad bowl, toss celery root with diced apples and lemon juice.

2. Cover the salad bowl with a plate for the time being.

3. In the meantime, in a small blender, blend cherries, dates, and grapefruit juice.

4. Spread the mix onto the celery and apples. Toss well to make sure the mix is evenly spread.

5. Now, top with some coconut cream, fresh mint, and crushed almonds. Enjoy!

*How to make your own vegan-friendly mayo:

Mix: ½ cup almond or coconut milk, 2 tablespoons fresh lemon juice, 1 tablespoon vegan mustard, half cup of olive oil, and a pinch of salt and pepper. You can experiment with the consistency by adding some almond powder and coconut oil. Enjoy!

Recipe #8 Kale Mixed Up Salad

In case you're wondering what scallions are, they are also known as green, spring, or salad onion. In this salad, they blend amazingly with kale to spice it up while offering a simple to make and healing alkaline salad.

Serves: 1-2

Ingredients:

- ½ cup of pistachios, shelled
- 1 cup of kale, chopped
- 4 scallions, thinly sliced

    + ¼ cup of raw sesame seeds (optional)

For the dressing:

- ¼ cup of tahini paste

- ¼ cup of coconut milk

- 1 garlic clove

- Himalayan salt, to taste

- Half a lemon, juiced

- 1 tablespoon miso paste

Instructions:

1.To prepare the salad dressing, blend all the ingredients until smooth. Add coconut milk to the dressing to achieve the right consistency.

2.Place the kale with scallions in a salad bowl.

3.Pour the salad dressing over the veggie mixture and toss well to combine. Try a piece of your salad to determine whether you need more salt and lemon juice to taste. If so, go ahead and add it now.

4.Finally, sprinkle the sesame seeds and the pistachios on top of the salad to garnish and serve the salad. Enjoy!

Recipe #9 Greek-Style Bell Pepper Salad

This salad will allow you to enjoy the taste of traditional Greek salad in a delicious plant-based version. You will also learn how to make your own vegan feta cheese (there is a bonus recipe at the end of the recipe). Still, it's up to you which option you decide to choose, or you may choose to leave it out.

Serves: 2

Ingredients:

- 1 large orange bell pepper (cut into bigger chunks)
- 1 large green bell pepper (cut into bigger chunks)
- 1 red bell pepper cut into chunks
- 1 cup of black olives, pitted
- 1 green onion, chopped
- ½ cup of organic walnuts, chopped
- 4 medium cucumbers, peeled and sliced
- ¼ cup parsley
- 1 cup of paleo cashew feta cheese, diced (optional) - Check the bonus recipe at the end!

Ingredients for the salad salsa:

- 2 tablespoons of olive oil (extra-virgin)
- 2 tablespoons of apple cider vinegar or Bragg Aminos
- 1 tablespoon of dried organic oregano

- 2 large garlic cloves, peeled and minced
- ½ teaspoon of Himalayan salt
- ½ teaspoon fresh black pepper

Instructions:

1. Start off by preparing the salad dressing by mixing all the ingredients for the vinaigrette in a small bowl or glass. Stir well with a fork.

2. Next, place all the vegetables into a salad bowl. Toss well. Add the feta cheese if you wish. Pour the salsa over the salad. Toss lightly to coat the vegetables with the vinaigrette.

3. You can serve the salad now or chill it for a few hours before serving.

***To make Vegan Paleo Cashew Feta-Style Cheese, simply blend the following ingredients:

- 1 cup of raw cashews soaked in water for at least a few hours (I leave it to soak overnight)
- About ¼ cup of almond milk or coconut milk
- 1 tablespoon of lime juice
- ¼ cup of nutritional yeast
- 1 clove of garlic and a bit of Himalayan salt to taste.

Transfer into ice cube trays and store in the fridge for a few hours.

Recipe #10 Gingered Pea Salad

Ginger is well-known for its anti-inflammatory and healing properties. And it's a fantastic ingredient to add to your soups, salads, and curries to spice them up.

Peas will add more substance to this salad. Cucumbers are highly refreshing and very alkaline-forming.

Serves: 2

Ingredients:

- 3 cucumbers, peeled and thinly sliced
- 1 tablespoon of grated ginger
- 2 tablespoons of coconut milk (thick) or coconut cream
- 1 tablespoon of raisins
- A few dates, pitted
- 2 green apples, sliced (optional- peeled)
- 2 tablespoons of fresh lemon juice
- ½ an avocado, sliced
- Black pepper to taste
- Himalayan salt to taste
- 3 tablespoons of sesame seeds

Instructions:

1.Place cucumbers, apples, and avocado in a salad bowl.

2.Pour over coconut milk and lemon juice. Toss well. Add sesame seeds and toss well again to distribute it evenly.

3.Season with Himalayan salt and black pepper and mix well. Add raisins and dates on top. Enjoy!

Recipe #11 Radish Wakame Salad

Wakame is a superfood. When I first heard about it a few years ago, I was attending workshops and classes about macrobiotic nutrition (always learning, always looking for information and always connecting with people who share the same passion for health), and I felt a bit frustrated. Not because I did not like it, but because it was very challenging to find it. Fortunately, the world is moving towards more healthy lifestyles. Those superfoods are getting more and more accessible! There are more health stores appearing every day, and even most supermarkets offer a range of original and lesser-known superfoods.

Wakame is very rich in magnesium, which is considered a highly alkaline-forming mineral.

If you can't find wakame, you can also use nori (same type of seaweed that is used for sushi). Then you just need to cut it into smaller pieces. The recipe will come out just as delicious. In fact, some people like it more with nori (sorry, my little Wakame, this recipe was supposed to be all about you and we are getting off topic now!). Experiment to see what works best for you.

Serves: 1-2

Ingredients:

- 1 whole cucumber, thinly sliced
- ½ cup of parsley, chopped
- 5 radishes, sliced

- 2 tablespoons of wakame seaweed, soaked in water as per instructions on the package
- Pinch of Himalayan salt, to taste (optional since usually wakame is already pretty salty)
- 2 tablespoons raw coconut vinegar
- ½ of a red onion, peeled and sliced thinly
- 1 tablespoon of olive oil (or grapeseed oil)
- 1 tablespoon orange juice, freshly squeezed
- Pinch of black pepper, to taste
- 2 orange wedges to garnish

Instructions:

1. Place cucumber, radish, parsley, onion, and wakame in a salad bowl.
2. In a separate bowl, add orange juice, olive or grapeseed oil, Himalayan salt, and black pepper. Mix well.
3. Pour onto your salad and toss well.
4. Serve with orange wedges and enjoy!

Recipe #12 Super-Quick Parsley Salad

It takes only a few of minutes to prepare, but you need much more time to drool over it!

Parsley is a miraculous ingredient, full of alkalizing properties. It's full of vitamins K, C, and E as well as iron to help you alkalize and take better care of your skin and eyes.

Servings: 1-2

Ingredients:

- 1 cup parsley leaves, chopped
- 2 tablespoons of cashews
- ½ cup cherry tomatoes
- 5 tablespoons of fresh pesto (simply blend some olive oil with Himalayan salt, fresh basil leaves, and tomato juice)
- 1 tablespoon chopped onion

Instructions:

1. Place parsley, cashew nuts, cherry tomato, and chopped onion into a salad bowl.
2. Poor over your fresh pesto.
3. Toss well and enjoy. Season with Himalayan salt if needed.

Recipe #13 Apple Pecan Tofu Salad

This salad offers a variety of plant-based protein mixed with the refreshing taste of apple and melon. It's easy to make and good for people who feel like eating an alkaline salad that is not green. When it comes to tofu, I am not the biggest fan of it. However, if you create a balanced diet, it's fine in moderation (organic, non-GMO tofu).

Serves:1-2

Ingredients:

- 1 can of smoked tofu, chopped
- 4 tablespoons of pecans
- 1 apple, diced
- ½ cup of lemon chunks
- ¼ cup coconut yogurt
- ½ stalk of celery, diced
- Ground black pepper, to taste
- ½ a lemon, juiced
- Himalayan salt, to taste
- A few mint leaves to garnish

Instructions:

1. Mix all the ingredients (aside from Himalayan salt and black pepper) in a salad bowl. Toss well.

2.Season with Himalayan salt and ground black pepper as needed.

3.Garnish with some fresh mint leaves. Enjoy!

Recipe #14 Quick Quinoa Salad

I love quinoa because it can be used in a variety of recipes and adapted to a variety of tastes. I also like it as it is an incredible natural source of protein and is all gluten-free (hence it's considered alkaline, because the alkaline diet and gluten do not go well together).

I like quinoa so much that I wrote a whole article about her on my blog (not too sure why I refer to quinoa as her):

www.HolisticWellnessProject.com/quinoa

Serves: 1-2

Ingredients:

- ½ cup cooked quinoa
- ¼ cup of radicchio (Italian chicory), shredded
- ¼ cup of raw walnuts, chopped
- 1 small and ripe avocado (peeled and diced)
- ¼ cup mixed leafy greens of your choice
- 2 tablespoons of vegan mayo
- 1 medium-sized endive, sliced
- 2 tablespoons of lemon juice
- 1 small seedless cucumber, diced
- ½ teaspoon of freshly cracked black pepper
- 1 teaspoon of herbs de Provence
- ¼ teaspoon of Himalayan or sea salt

- 2 tablespoons of olive oil

Instructions:

1.Simply place all the salad ingredients into a salad. Mix well.

2.Add a bit of vegan mayo and stir well.

3.Season the salad with Himalayan salt, pepper, olive oil, and lemon juice. Toss well to combine.

4.Enjoy!

Recipe #15 Arugula Lentil Salad with Lemon Parsley Dressing

This salad offers an incredible mix of clean, plant-based protein from lentils and iron backed up with vitamin C from the orange. And it's all nicely blended in an original dressing that tastes delicious!

Serves: 2

Ingredients:

- ½ cup of cooked lentils, cooled down
- 1 whole scallion, finely chopped
- 4 cups of fresh arugula, chopped
- 1 orange, peeled and sliced
- Fresh chopped parsley for topping
- 1 ripe avocado, peeled, pitted, and cubed
- 2 tablespoons of guacamole (optional)
- 1 tablespoon coconut milk
- 1 tablespoon olive oil

For the dressing:

- 2 tablespoons of extra virgin olive oil
- 4 tablespoons of parsley, chopped
- 2 tablespoons organic lemon juice

- 2 pinches of Himalayan salt (you can always add more if you need to)
- A pinch of pepper
- Lemon or lime wedges for garnishing

Instructions:

1. Place all the salad ingredients in a salad bowl. Mix well.

2. In a separate bowl, place all the ingredients for the dressing. Stir well.

3. Finally, pour the dressing into the salad bowl and toss well. Garnish with some lime or lemon wedges. Enjoy!

Recipe #16 Olive Creation Salad

This salad is a great solution if you are looking for a meal replacing salad, something that will keep you full for many hours. It's a great mix of veggies, protein, and good carbs from cooked sweet potatoes. It will spice up your lunch time for sure, at it's one of my favorite takeaway lunches. Enjoy!

Serves: 1-2

Ingredients:

- ½ cup black beans, cooked
- 1 cup of fresh cherry tomatoes
- Half cup black olives, pitted
- A few tablespoon of green olives
- 2 whole medium sweet potatoes (boiled and cooled)
- 1 cucumber, peeled and finely chopped
- A few onion rings
- Handful of fresh baby spinach leaves
- A pinch (or 2) of garlic powder

For dressing:

- 3 tablespoons of Dijon mustard
- ½ tablespoon of organic olive oil
- Sea salt to taste

- 1 tablespoon of coconut vinegar
- Black pepper to taste

Instructions:

1. Simply place all the salad ingredients in a salad bowl. Mix well.

2. Now proceed to creating the salad dressing by mixing all the ingredients in a separate salad bowl. Stir well.

3. Now, pour the salad dressing over your salad and enjoy.

4. If you are planning to use this recipe as a take away lunch, I suggest you save your salad dressing in a separate small container and mix it with your salad when you're ready to devour it. Yeah, it's that tasty (and so simple to make!).

Recipe #17 Coconut Chickpeas with Roasted Broccoli Salad

This salad offers a unique mix of roasted broccoli, chickpeas, and a ton of veggies.

While this salad might take a while to make, it's definitely worth it. For me, it's a perfect comfort salad for dinner, and the leftovers can be used for a quick brunch or lunch the next day.

Servings: 1-2

Ingredients:

- 2 cups of broccoli, chopped into florets
- ½ cup of green olives
- ½ cup chickpeas
- 1 tablespoon of coconut oil
- ½ teaspoon curry powder
- ½ of an avocado, peeled and sliced
- ½ cup of cherry tomatoes, quartered
- Handful of almonds
- A pinch of sea salt
- 1 tablespoon of vegan mustard
- 1 tablespoon of olive oil
- 1-2 oz. of vegan feta cheese, diced (Optional)
- Black pepper, to taste

Instructions:

1. First, place the broccoli florets into a baking dish and drizzle over some olive oil.

2. Add the dried garlic, salt, and black pepper to the broccoli florets (you can also add other spices of your choice, like oregano, but this is optional).

3. Now, toss the broccoli florets with the added ingredients and transfer to a 400 degrees Fahrenheit (200 Celsius) preheated oven. Roast for 30-35 minutes.

4. In the meantime, stir-fry the chickpeas in some coconut oil and curry powder (half teaspoon) and Himalayan salt. Use low heat. It should take about 10 minutes.

5. As you keep an eye on your chickpeas and broccoli, place green olives, avocado, cherry tomatoes, almonds, a pinch of Himalayan salt, Dijon mustard, olive oil, vegan feta cheese, and black pepper in a salad bowl. Stir well. Cover and place in the fridge.

6. Check the chickpeas, they should be slightly crunchy now. Turn off the heat and cool them down.

7. When ready, take out the cooled roasted broccoli and add it to your salad. Do the same with stir-fried chickpeas. Stir well again and enjoy!

Recipe #18 Smoked Tofu and Sweet Potato Green Salad

This salad offers another filling lunch option while combining all the alkaline benefits of veggies, natural plant-based protein, and good carbs (and sweetness!) from sweet potatoes. Horseradish cream spices it up and gives it a unique flavor.

This salad is perfect as a takeaway lunch that will keep you full until the late afternoon or early evening.

Serves: 1-2

Ingredients:

- ½ cup of smoked tofu, cut into smaller pieces
- 3 large sweet potatoes, cooked, diced, and cooled down
- 1 teaspoon of horseradish cream
- 1 large organic tomato, sliced
- 1 small cucumber, peeled and sliced
- ½ cup coconut yogurt
- 1 cup fresh watercress
- Juice of 1 lemon
- A dash of ground black pepper
- Himalayan salt to taste

Instructions:

1. Place all the ingredients into a salad bowl. Stir well.

2. Season with black pepper and Himalayan salt to taste.

3. Enjoy!

Recipe #19 Artichoke Dream

Artichokes are highly alkalizing and full of magnesium and potassium.

They're the perfect ingredient for a healing, refreshing green alkaline salad like this one!

Serves: 1-2

Ingredients:

- 1 cup of canned artichoke hearts, halved
- 1 cup of fresh kale leaves, stemmed and coarsely chopped
- 1 kiwi, peeled and sliced
- ½ a red onion, sliced
- ½ cup coconut yoghurt
- 2 tablespoons of lime juice
- 2 slices of lime to garnish
- Handful of cashews to garnish
- Handful of cilantro to garnish
- Pinch of Himalayan salt to taste

Instructions:

1. Mix all of the salad ingredients in a large bowl.
2. Stir well while adding the coconut yogurt.

3.Season with Himalayan salt. Garnish with cashews, cilantro, and limes slices. Enjoy!

Recipe #20 Avocado Dream Salad

This salad is great for a quick, highly alkalizing snack! Avocado is full of good fats and for long-term diet success. And just like coconut oil, it helps prevent sugar cravings. Enjoy!

Serves: 1-2

Ingredients:

- 4 tablespoons of cooked chickpeas
- 4 tablespoons of cooked quinoa
- 1 whole avocado
- A Pinch of black pepper to taste
- 1 large fresh organic tomato, diced
- A pinch of sea salt to taste
- 1 lime, juiced
- Handful of cilantro, to taste and for garnish

Instructions

1. Simply place all the ingredients in a salad bowl and stir well.
2. Garnish with cilantro and enjoy!

Recipe #21 Curry Love Quinoa Salad

This salad takes advantage of the anti-inflammatory benefits of curry spice while sneaking in some greens full of alkaline benefits and a unique taste combination thanks to grapes.

Serves: 1-2

Ingredients:

- ½ cup cooked quinoa
- 1 cup radicchio
- Handful of walnut halves
- 2 tablespoons of vegan mayonnaise
- 1 cup of red grapes, halved
- 2 tablespoons of coconut vinegar
- 1 large celery rib, halved lengthwise and thinly sliced crosswise
- ¼ cup of mixed baby greens
- 1 teaspoon of curry powder
- ½ teaspoon of black pepper
- Himalayan salt to season

Instructions:

1.Place all the ingredients in a large salad bowl and stir well.

2.Season with some Himalayan salt and serve right away or cool down in the fridge for a few hours.

3.Enjoy!

Recipe #22 Tofu Salad with Mango and Avocado

Salads are not boring! There is always room for creativity. Personally, I love experimenting with a small amount of fruit in my salads. For this recipe, I chose mango. Tofu can be replaced with any other protein of your choice.

Serves: 1-2

Ingredients:

- 2 tablespoons of mango chutney
- ½ cup chopped smoked tofu (organic, not genetically modified)
- 1 cup of mixed salad greens
- 1 tablespoon of olive oil or grapeseed oil
- 1 cup of peeled and diced mango
- 2 tablespoons of fresh lime juice
- 1 small avocado, peeled and diced
- 1 tablespoon of coconut aminos
- 1 teaspoon of grated fresh ginger
- A handful of raisins and cashews to garnish
- Pinch of Himalayan salt to taste

Instructions:

1. Place all the ingredients into a salad bowl.

2. Pour over olive or grapeseed oil, lime juice, and coconut aminos.

3. Stir well.

4. Season with Himalayan salt.

5. Sprinkle over some raisins and cashews to garnish.

6. Serve fresh and enjoy!

Recipe #23 Holiday Cranberry Buckwheat Salad

Buckwheat is one of those incredible gluten-free grains which makes it a perfect ingredient for an alkaline salad!

Buckwheat is full of magnesium and manganese, which are super-alkaline minerals. At the same time, it's a healthy source of carbohydrates.

Cranberries bring in some unique flavor here and spice the salad up!

Serves: 1-2

Ingredients:

- 1 cup of cooked buckwheat, cooled down
- 1 cup of celery, chopped
- 1 cup of chopped pecans
- 4 tablespoons of vegan mayonnaise (preferably homemade)
- Himalayan salt, to taste
- ½ cup of minced green bell pepper
- 1 cup of cranberries
- 1 fresh green onion, chopped
- 1 teaspoon of paprika
- Ground black pepper, to taste
- 2 tablespoons lemon juice
- 1 tablespoon olive oil

Instructions:

1. Place all the ingredients in a salad bowl.

2. Mix well to ensure all the ingredients are equally seasoned.

3. Serve right away and enjoy or store in the fridge for later.

Recipe #24 Mediterranean Cilantro Chickpea Salad

Not only is cilantro highly alkalizing, it also brings some unique flavor to this salad!

Chickpeas add natural protein while veggies help restore energy levels due to high levels of alkaline minerals.

Serves: 1-2

Ingredients:

- ½ cup chickpeas, cooked, drained, and cooled
- A few leaves of romaine lettuce, chopped
- Half a lemon, juiced
- 4 tablespoons of fresh cilantro, roughly chopped
- ½ a red onion, diced
- 1 small red bell pepper, chopped
- 1 cucumber, peeled and chopped
- 1 clove of garlic
- ½ an avocado, peeled and sliced
- 4 tablespoons of coconut cream
- Pinch of Himalayan salt to taste
- Black pepper to taste

Instructions:

1. Place all the ingredients into a salad bowl, adding lemon juice, coconut cream, Himalayan salt, and black pepper.

2. Serve right away or store in a fridge and serve slightly chilled.

3. Enjoy!

Recipe #25 Coconut Quinoa Salad

Sometimes, you may find plain quinoa boring or even tasteless. That is why I created this recipe, because it makes quinoa exciting and fun! Nothing tastes as good as coconut quinoa spiced up with garlic, anti-inflammatory spices, and served with some greens and good fats from avocado (very alkaline-forming).

Serves: 1-2

Ingredients:

- 1 cup of cooked quinoa
- ¼ cup vegan broth of your choice
- 2 tablespoons fresh lime juice
- ¼ cup of mint leaves
- ¼ cup chopped cilantro leaves
- Handful of raisins
- Himalayan salt to taste
- 1 small avocado, peeled, pitted, and sliced
- 2 tablespoons of coconut oil
- 2 garlic cloves
- 1 teaspoon cumin powder (feel free to use less if you don't like it spicy)
- 1 teaspoon curry powder (feel free to use less if you don't like it spicy)

- ½ cup cherry tomatoes

Instructions:

1. Place coconut oil into a small frying pan and heat up over medium heat. Add chopped garlic, stir well, and then add quinoa and a pinch of Himalayan salt.

2. Keep stir-frying and add the spices.

3. Now, as you keep stir-frying, slowly add in the vegan broth. The best moment to do so is when you notice that your frying pan is "running out" of coconut oil.

4. Increase the heat a little bit. Keep stir-frying until the quinoa has completely absorbed the spices and the vegan broth.

5. Turn off the heat and set aside. Let the quinoa cool down in the fridge.

6. In the meantime, place the cilantro and mint leaves into a medium salad bowl.

7. On one side, place the sliced avocado and cherry tomatoes.

8. On the other side, place the cooked and cooled quinoa.

9. Sprinkle over some raisins and pour over some fresh lime juice. It adds a twist to this salad.

10. Serve now or cool down in the fridge.

Suggestion: If you want to make it a solid, plant-based protein lunch bowl, then add some chickpeas as well. Enjoy!

Recipe #26 Hazelnut Banana Salad

This salad is incredible if you are craving something sweet. While not strictly alkaline (bananas are a sugary fruit), it is an excellent, healthy alternative to satisfy your sweet tooth without compromising your health.

Serves: 1-2

Ingredients:

- ½ cup hazelnuts
- 1 banana, sliced
- 1 cup strawberries, halved
- ½ cup coconut milk (preferably thick)
- ½ teaspoon of maca powder
- 2 tablespoons raw cocoa
- Handful of raisins

Instructions:

1. Place hazelnuts, banana, and strawberries into a salad bowl.
2. In another bowl, add coconut milk, cocoa powder, and maca. Stir well. You can also use a blender.
3. Next, add this mixture to your fruit salad. Stir well.
4. Sprinkle over some raisins to taste.
5. Serve now or store in the fridge to serve cooled.
6. Enjoy!

Recipe #27 Roasted Asparagus Salad

This is an incredible low-carb alkaline salad that offers a unique taste thanks to its vinaigrette. Enjoy!

Serves: 1-2

Ingredients:

- 1 cup chickpeas, cooked and cooled
- 1 whole ripe avocado, peeled pitted and sliced
- ½ cup of asparagus, chopped into 2-3 inch pieces
- ½ cup of baby spinach leaves, chopped
- 2 tablespoons coconut oil

For the alkaline vinaigrette:

- 2 tablespoons of olive oil
- 1 teaspoon of vegan mustard
- 2 tablespoons of coconut vinegar
- 2 teaspoons of rosemary, finely chopped
- 1 large clove garlic (peeled and minced)
- 1 tablespoon of thyme, minced
- ½ teaspoon of black pepper
- A pinch of Himalayan salt
- Half a lemon, juiced

Instructions:

1. Stir-fry chickpeas in coconut oil (medium heat). Add a pinch of Himalayan salt to taste.

2. Chop the asparagus and add to the same pan over the chickpea drippings. Stir-fry the asparagus for 4-5 minutes or until the asparagus gets imbued with the coconut flavors. Turn off the heat once done and set the pan aside.

3. Next, throw all the ingredients for the vinaigrette into a small bowl or glass jar and whisk with a metal whisk to make the vinaigrette.

4. Place the baby spinach leaves into a salad bowl and add the chickpeas and asparagus.

5. Now, add the avocado slices as well and drizzle a little bit of vinaigrette on top.

6. Stir well and serve immediately.

Recipe #28 Kiwi Spinach Lentil Energizer

This salad offers a very smart combination: Iron from spinach and lentils (which also provide protein, which is crucial to keep you energized) with vitamin C from kiwis. It's all you need to help your body absorb this precious Iron better and faster so that you can feel energized and happy.

Serves: 1-2

Ingredients:

- 1 cup organic lentils, soaked and cooked
- 2 whole kiwis, peeled and sliced
- 4 tablespoons of raisins
- A few strawberries, halved
- ¼ cup fresh baby spinach
- 2 tablespoons of organic apple juice
- Himalayan salt, to taste
- Black pepper, to taste
- 1 tablespoon lemon juice
- 1 cucumber, sliced
- 2 tablespoons grapeseed or olive oil

Instructions:

1. Place lentils, spinach, cucumber, and kiwis into a salad bowl. Mix well.

2. Pour over some lemon juice, apple juice, and grapeseed or olive oil.

3. Finally, add some Himalayan salt, black pepper, and raisins. Toss well.

4. Garnish with some strawberries, serve fresh, and enjoy!

Recipe #29 Green Spicy Salad

We all know greens are good for us. But how do we make greens easy, exciting, and fun? Well, this salad offers all the answers! Plus, spices are very alkalizing and full of anti-inflammatory benefits. That is what it's all about.

Serves: 1-2

Ingredients for the salsa:

- 2 cloves of garlic, minced
- 1 tablespoon of olive oil
- A pinch of ground cumin
- 2 tablespoons of fresh lemon juice
- 2 tablespoons coconut milk
- 1 teaspoon curry powder
- ¾ teaspoon of fine-grain sea salt
- ¼ teaspoon of ground coriander

Salad:

- ½ cup of fresh spring greens
- 2 handfuls of fresh basil leaves, torn roughly
- 2 handfuls of fresh cherry tomatoes, cut in halves
- 1 whole avocado, peeled, pitted, and sliced
- Handful of fresh parsley, stemmed and chopped

Instructions:

1. First, blend all of the salsa ingredients and set aside.
2. Next, place all the salad ingredients into a medium-sized salad bowl. Mix well.
3. Pour over the salsa, stir well, and enjoy. Serve fresh!

Recipe #30 Buckwheat Salad with Spinach

Could it be so simple? Yes, health is not that hard. One alkaline salad a day can absolutely keep the doctor away. Simplicity is the key to success. I love this salad when I am pressed for time. You can use buckwheat leftovers, or swap buckwheat for quinoa.

Despite its name, buckwheat is not wheat. It's gluten-free and more than compatible with the alkaline diet (unless you don't like it for some reason, and if that's the case, perhaps this recipe will make you change your mind).

Serves: 1-2

Ingredients:

- ½ cup of fresh strawberries, sliced
- 1 cup of fresh baby spinach
- ½ cup buckwheat, cooked and chilled
- Handful of chopped almonds
- A handful of raisins to garnish

Dressing:

- 1 tablespoon of coconut vinegar
- 2 tablespoons of olive oil
- 2 tablespoons of fresh lemon juice
- 1 teaspoon of Dijon mustard

- 1 teaspoon of raw honey
- Pinch of black pepper
- Pinch of Himalayan salt, to taste

Instructions:

1. Whisk all the dressing ingredients until they become smooth and well-combined.

2. Combine the spinach with almonds, strawberries, and buckwheat, then drizzle the prepared dressing over the salad.

3. Toss the salad lightly to mix well, garnish with raisins, and serve immediately. Enjoy!

Recipe #31 Watermelon Salad with Pecans and Cherries

This salad offers a very smart way of sneaking in some greens. Perfect for beginners who still are having hard time with veggies. Why not fruit it up? Oh, and there is also some ginger, which helps your immune system and is well-known for its anti-inflammatory properties.

Serves: 1-2

Ingredients:

- ½ cup of pecans, lightly toasted and chopped
- 1 head of butterhead (Boston) lettuce, chopped
- 1 teaspoon of grated ginger, fresh
- 1 cup watermelon, chopped
- ½ cup of dried cherries, pitted
- ⅓ cup of coconut yogurt
- A pinch of sea salt
- 1 lime, juiced

Instructions:

1. Place all the ingredients into a salad bowl.

2. Mix well and enjoy! You can serve it now or cool it down in the fridge for a couple of hours. Perfect for hot summers, as a snack, or for a light and healthy dessert.

Recipe #32 Plant-Based Greek Salad

This super-tasty Greek salad can be easily made in a plant-based, lactose-free version with vegan Paleo Cashew Feta-style cheese.

Serves: 1-2

Ingredients:

- 1 cup of chopped romaine lettuce
- ½ cup of crumbled paleo feta cheese*** (Optional, just follow the recipe below)
- 2 tablespoons of coconut vinegar
- 2 medium-sized tomatoes, chopped
- 2 tablespoons of olive oil (extra-virgin)
- ½ cup of sliced ripe black olives
- 1 tablespoon of fresh dill, chopped
- 1 large cucumber, peeled and chopped
- 1 teaspoon of garlic powder
- ¼ teaspoon Himalayan salt
- 1 small onion, chopped
- A pinch of freshly-ground pepper

How to Make Vegan Paleo Cashew Feta-Style Cheese:

Blend:

-1 cup of raw cashews soaked in water for at least a few hours (I leave them to soak overnight)

-About ¼ cup of almond milk or coconut milk

-1 tablespoon of lime juice

-¼ cup of nutritional yeast

-1 clove of garlic and a bit of Himalayan salt to taste.

-Transfer into ice cube trays or square molds and store in the fridge for a few hours.

Instructions:

1. Place the olives, romaine lettuce, paleo feta cheese, cucumber, onions, and tomatoes into a salad bowl. Toss well.

2. In a separate bowl, whisk the olive oil, coconut vinegar, dill, ground black pepper, and sea salt into a bowl.

3. Now, pour the dressing over the salad and toss again before serving. Enjoy!

Recipe #33 Summer Veggie Color Salad

Beetroot is an incredible salad addition and is considered a very alkalizing food. It blends well with the rest of the veggies and tastes amazing, especially when served with our alkaline-friendly fresh parsley salad dressing!

Serves: 1-2

Ingredients:

- 6 whole radishes, sliced
- 1 beetroot, peeled and sliced
- ½ of a red onion, peeled and sliced
- 1 small zucchini, sliced and lightly cooked
- 1 small kohlrabi, sliced
- 1 red pepper, deseeded and sliced
- ¼ cup of cashews

Alkaline Salad Dressing:

- 2 tablespoons of olive oil (extra virgin)
- 2 teaspoons of fresh oregano, chopped
- 1 clove of garlic, peeled and finely chopped
- 1 tablespoon of fresh parsley leaves, chopped
- 2 tablespoons of water
- Juice of 1 fresh lemon

- A pinch of sea salt

Instructions:

1. First, mix all of the alkaline salad dressing ingredients. Whisk well.

2. Now, mix the salad veggies in a large salad bowl. Add some cashews and drizzle the alkaline salad dressing on top to serve the salad.

3. Enjoy!

Recipe #34 Green Papaya Dream Salad

Papaya is fantastic for digestive wellness and combines amazingly with veggies. This is another great example of a simple "beginner salad" where you can easily squeeze in some greens and enjoy the combination while taking care of your body and mind to stay energized.

Servings: 1-2

Ingredients:

- ¼ cup of mixed fresh lettuce leaves
- ½ of a green papaya, julienned
- ¼ cup radish, sliced
- 1 carrot, spiralized
- 2 tablespoons of chia seeds
- A few whole cherry tomatoes, sliced

For the Spicy Chili Dressing:

- 1 tablespoon of raw coconut vinegar
- 5 dates, pitted
- 2 tablespoons of water
- 1 red long chili, seeded and finely chopped
- Juice of 2 limes
- 2 tablespoons of vegan vegetable broth

- 1 small clove of garlic, peeled and minced
- Pinch of Himalayan salt

Instructions:

1. First, blend all of the ingredients for the Chili Spicy Dressing.

2. Place all of the salad ingredients into a large salad bowl and mix well.

3. Finaly, pour over the Spicy Chili Dressing. Toss well and enjoy!

Recipe #35 Green Orange Salad

Yes, I can hear the confusion out there, but this salad is clearly not about green oranges. It's about mixing oranges with greens to take advantage of vitamin C (which oranges are rich in) and chlorophyll (found in greens) to help you detoxify your body and stay energized. Use this salad as a snack and there will be no unwanted food cravings nor feeling tired and like you need another cup of coffee.

Serves: 2

Ingredients:

- 3 whole fresh oranges, peeled and sliced
- 5 tablespoons of coconut cream or any plant-based yoghurt of your choice (sugar-free)
- 2 cups of mixed Asian greens
- 3 tablespoons of coconut vinegar
- 1 red bell pepper, seeded and chopped
- ½ teaspoon of five-spice powder, organic
- ½ cup of slivered red onion
- Pinch of Himalayan salt
- A pinch of freshly-ground black pepper

Instructions:

1.Place oranges, Asian greens, red bell pepper, and onion into a medium-sized salad bowl. Mix well.

2.Now pour over the coconut cream and coconut vinegar.

3.Sprinkle over the spices and some salt. Stir well and enjoy!

Recipe #36 Yummy Grilled Zucchini Salad

This is a fantastic recipe for a family barbecue or for those days when you get tired eating raw foods. To be quite honest with you, this recipe is one of my favorite comfort foods. And it's one of those guilt-free comfort foods, so enjoy!

Serves: 1-2

Ingredients:

- 2 whole fresh zucchini, quartered lengthwise
- 1 cup of cherry tomatoes, quartered or halved
- 2 tablespoons of sweet onion, minced
- 2 teaspoons of olive oil (extra virgin)
- 20 black olives, pitted and roughly chopped
- A pinch of crushed garlic
- 1 tablespoon of fresh lemon thyme
- 1 tablespoon of fresh dill, chopped
- 1 teaspoon of Dijon mustard (optional)
- A pinch of Himalayan salt
- ¼ teaspoon black pepper
- Juice of ½ a lemon
- 1-2 tablespoons of avocado or coconut oil
- Sea salt, to taste
- Black pepper, to taste

Instructions:

1. First, toss the zucchini in 2 tablespoons of olive oil, salt, garlic, and a bit of black pepper.

2. Set aside and allow the zucchini slices to marinate for 10 minutes.

3. Grill over medium heat after marinating until the zucchini slices are slightly blackened.

4. Remove from the grill and let the zucchini slices cool down.

5. As it's cooling down, mix some olive oil with Dijon mustard and lemon juice. Stir well.

6. Add the cherry tomatoes, olives, and sweet onions to the zucchini.

7. Toss the vegetables with the olive oil-mustard mixture from step 5.

8. Finally, add the herbs and toss again. Serve and enjoy!

Recipe #37 Happy Mizeria Salad

The reason why I call this salad a "Happy Mizeria" salad is very simple: it's inspired by a Polish salad recipe called Mizeria. Which, for English speakers, might be close to "misery," which is definitely not my intention. I promote wellness, not misery. That being said, it's a very tasty and refreshing salad that, when created in its alkaline version (just like the recipe below), is fully plant-based and full of alkaline healing benefits.

Serves: 1-2

Ingredients:

- 4 large cucumbers
- ½ an onion, peeled and cut into rings
- ½ cup radish, sliced
- ½ cup coconut cream
- Handful of cashews
- Himalayan salt to taste
- ¼ teaspoon of black pepper
- 1 tablespoon lemon juice

Instructions:

1. Mix all of the salad ingredients in a salad bowl
2. Add coconut cream, salt, and pepper.

3.Stir well and sprinkle over some lemon juice, stir again.

4.Serve right away or place in the fridge to serve later. Enjoy!

Recipe #38 Fennel Salad with Tahini Coconut Dressing

I am not new to juicing fennel. In fact, it appears frequently in my juicing recipes on my blog and in my book Alkaline Juicing. However, fennel in salads is something new to me. I have good news though. I have been running some experiments, and I can tell you one thing: even if you are new to this, it will taste great.

Serves: 2-3

Ingredients for the salad:

- 3 heads of fennel, cored and thinly sliced
- A handful of raisins
- ¼ cup of iceberg lettuce
- ¼ cup of Thai basil
- 1 whole red bell pepper, seeded and sliced
- Handful of cashews to garnish

Ingredients for the dressing:

- 4 tablespoons of fresh coconut milk
- 4 tablespoons of tahini
- 1 inch of fresh ginger, grated (or 1-2 teaspoons of ginger powder)
- 1 teaspoon of almond butter

- Juice of 1 lime
- Pinch of Himalayan salt
- Pinch of black pepper

Instructions:

1. Place all the salad ingredients into a bowl. Mix well.
2. In a separate salad bowl, add all the dressing ingredients and whisk well.
3. Pour the salad dressing over the salad.
4. Garnish with some cashews, serve, and enjoy!

Bonus: Healthy Alkaline Salad Sauces and Condiments

While I have already introduced you to many healthy alkaline friendly salsas and salad dressings in this book, I wanted to add a few more so that you can enjoy more variety. Even the most boring salads get tasty again as long as you spice them up with interesting and creative dressings. I hope you enjoy this bonus section!

Simple Alkaline Tahini Salad Dressing

Servings: 1-2 (¼ cup)

Ingredients:

- 2-3 tablespoons of Tahini (sesame seed butter)
- Organic apple cider vinegar, to taste
- 2 cloves of garlic
- Sea salt, to taste
- 1 lemon, juiced
- Ground black pepper, to taste

Instructions:

1. Simply blend all the ingredients until well-combined and smooth.
2. Add more water or apple cider vinegar to loosen the dressing if required.

Almost Alkaline Orange Dressing

I love this dressing not only for salads, but also for guilt-free sweet potato fries! Yes, we can make our own "fast food" in a healthier alkaline version.

Servings: 2

Ingredients:

- 1 tablespoon of vegan mustard
- 1 orange, juiced
- 1 tablespoon of poppy seeds (can be replaced with chia seeds)
- Zest of 1 orange
- 1 garlic clove, smashed
- 1 teaspoon of coconut vinegar
- 4 tablespoons of vegan mayonnaise
- ¼ teaspoon of ground white pepper
- ¼ teaspoon of Himalayan salt

Instructions:

1. Blend all the ingredients until you achieve smooth salad dressing.
2. Serve with an alkaline salad of your choice and enjoy!

Chive Salad Dressing

This is one of my favorite salad dressings because it blends well with most of my salads. It also offers a variety of good oils.

Servings: 2

Ingredients:

- 1 tablespoon of hemp oil
- ½ teaspoon of maple syrup
- 1 teaspoon of coconut vinegar
- 1 tablespoon of finely-chopped chives
- 1 clove fresh garlic, minced
- 1 tablespoon of grapeseed oil

Instructions:

1. Combine all of the ingredients in a bowl.
2. Whisk the mixture until everything is well-combined. Serve with an alkaline salad of your choice!

Alkaline Carrot Ginger Salad Dressing

Servings: 6

Ingredients:

- ¼ cup of peeled and chopped carrots,
- 4 tablespoons of apple cider vinegar
- 1 tablespoon of coconut aminos
- ¼ cup of fresh ginger, peeled and chopped
- 2 tablespoons hemp or grapeseed oil
- ½ an onion, chopped
- ⅛ teaspoon of Himalayan salt
- 1 tablespoon of sesame oil
- 1 lemon, juiced

Instructions:

1. Blend all the ingredients in a hand blender.
2. Add some water if needed and blend again.
3. Serve with an alkaline salad of your choice. Enjoy!

Creamy Citrus Dressing

This is a very simple and original dressing that can also be used as a garnish.

Servings: 1

Ingredients:

- 2 tablespoons of fresh orange juice
- 1 teaspoon of organic almond butter or any other nut butter
- Himalayan salt, to taste
- 1 tablespoon of avocado or grapeseed oil
- Pinch of black pepper, to taste
- ¼ teaspoon of minced garlic

Instructions:

1. Mix all the ingredients in a small salad bowl and whisk well.
2. Serve with an alkaline salad of your choice.

Italian-Style Tomato Cilantro Dressing

Honestly, I am addicted to Italian flavors and spices. You can still enjoy that taste while creating healthy and alkaline salads!

Servings: 4

Ingredients:

- 1 large tomato, peeled
- 4 tablespoons of olive oil
- 2 cloves of garlic, peeled
- ½ small red onion
- A handful of fresh cilantro
- 1 green onion
- Sea salt, to taste
- Black pepper, to taste

Instructions:

1. Blend all the ingredients in a blender. Make sure everything is smooth.

2. Serve with a yummy alkaline salad of your choice!

Catalina Almost-Alkaline Dressing

Spicy dressings like this one can make even a bowl of lettuce or kale more exciting and fun (and tasty!).

Servings: 1 cup

Ingredients:

- 2 tablespoons of fresh tomato paste
- 6 tablespoons of olive oil
- 1 teaspoon of vegan mustard
- 4 tablespoons of raw apple cider vinegar
- ½ teaspoon of paprika
- 1 tablespoon of maple syrup
- ½ teaspoon of garlic powder
- ¼ teaspoon of chili powder
- A pinch of black pepper

Instructions:

1. Place all of the ingredients into a salad bowl and whisk well.
2. Serve with an alkaline salad of your choice and enjoy!

Creating Your Alkaline Lifestyle for Energy You Deserve

Take meaningful and purposeful action today. You already know that you need to add more alkaline foods into your diet. That does not mean that you should live on salads alone. It just means that you should be committed to pursuing alkalinity by adding more living alkaline foods into your diet, alkaline salads included. Here are a few simple steps that you can implement to feel more energized in a week or less. Of course, the more you do, the better for you.

-Try to have at least 1 large salad a day. You can also start adding more greens to your other meals. Again, this does not mean that you should live on greens and green salads alone. But you should get in a habit of serving massive portions of leafy green veggies with your meals.

-Drink plenty of filtered alkaline water. You can purchase a water pitcher, which will save you money in the long run. Most bottled water brands have an acidifying effect on our body. Switching to alkaline water will be the best health investment you have ever made. Going alkaline does not mean you have to go 100% vegan (of course you can, and I will support your decision). However, it does encourage you to reduce your consumption of animal products. There are many other plant-based options that are better for the environment and your health. Also, looking for more vegan options (even if you are not vegan) stimulates creativity.

-Reduce caffeine. As soon as you start adding more alkaline foods into your diet, your energy levels will skyrocket.

-Ask yourself every day how you can add more veggies, especially raw ones, into your diet.

-Move your body. If you are not a gym person, start going for long revitalizing walks. Ask a friend to accompany you if you feel like that will help you get and stay motivated. You can also combine your walks with your social life. Just call a friend or create a health group via meetup.com.

-Relax, practice mindfulness, and live in the NOW. Most of our "Western society" problems are nothing compared to what people in other countries experience. We have everything. We should be grateful, not complaining. Keep in mind that the alkaline diet lifestyle is not only about what you eat and drink. It's also about how you live and what you think. I have a free guided meditation recording you can get at: holisticwellnessproject.com/meditation

-Spend more time embracing your hobbies and things you enjoy doing. It doesn't have to be anything professional. Just follow your passion and personal fulfillment.

For more wellness inspiration and empowerment visit:

www.alkalinedietlifestyle.com

www.holisticwellnessproject.com

Don't forget to grab your 3 free Alkaline Diet eBooks:

www.holisticwellnessproject.com/alkaline

Marta's Holistic Wellness Books

I have written many more books related to wellness, the alkaline diet, living a healthy lifestyle, and motivation. They are available as eBooks, paperbacks, and some even as audiobooks for your convenience.

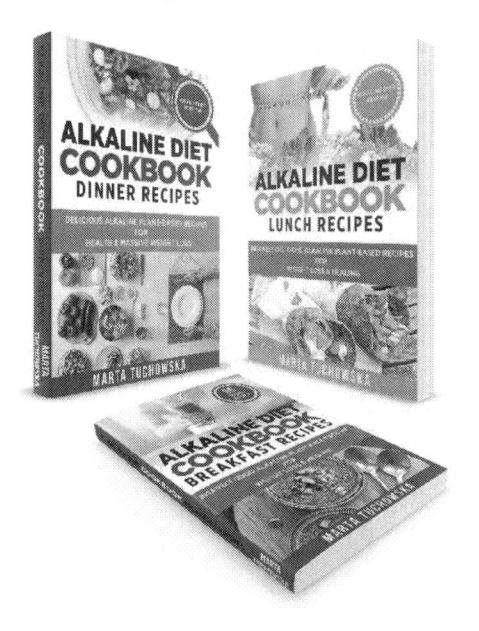

The most popular of my books are "Alkaline Smoothies," "Alkaline Smoothie Bowls," and "How to Lose Massive Weight with the Alkaline Diet." You will also find many other books of my authorship such as "Alkaline Juicing," "Alkaline Drinks," and "Alkaline Diet Motivation."

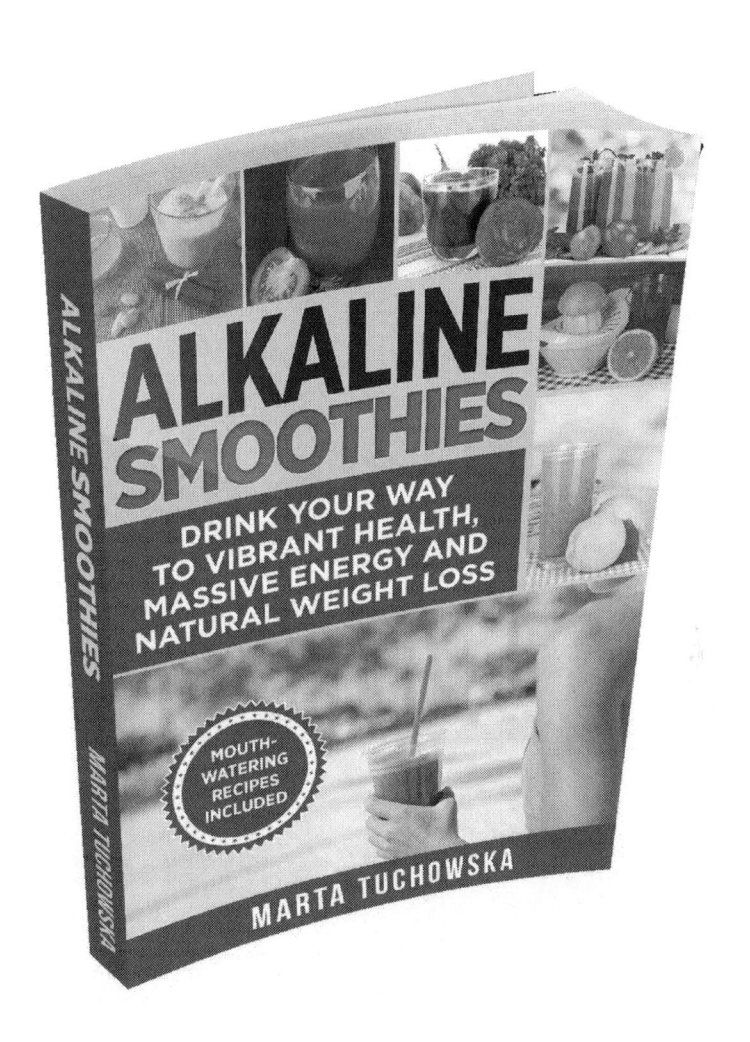

You will find all of my books by exploring the links below:

www.holisticwellnessproject.com/alkaline-diet-books

www.holisticwellnessproject.com/books

I have been passionately and actively researching, living, teaching, and writing about this lifestyle since 2013.

You will also find a ton of extra information on my blog:

www.HolisticWellnessProject.com

Thanks again for your time and interest in my work.

It was a pleasure to "talk" to you,

I hope we "meet" again soon!

Marta "Wellness" Tuchowska (I realize that my surname is not the easiest to remember, but "Marta Wellness" is fine)

In the meantime, let's connect:

www.instagram.com/Marta_Wellness

www.facebook.com/HolisticWellnessProject

www.twitter.com/Marta_Wellness

Do not forget to follow my Amazon Author profile to be notified about my new books at discounted launch prices and giveaways:

www.amazon.com/author/mtuchowska

You can also join my insider Alkaline Wellness Newsletter at:

www.HolisticWellnessProject.com/alkaline and unlock 3 free bonus eBooks (alkaline diet and recipes).

I wish you wellness, health, and success in whatever you want to accomplish.

Marta

P.S. Before you go, could you please do something for me? If you received any value from this book, could you please post a short review and let others know about your experience? It will help more readers take better care of their health and enjoy the healing benefits of alkaline salads and healthy foods in general. It will only take a few seconds. It's you that I am writing for, and I would love to hear from you in the review section of this book!

Printed in Great Britain
by Amazon